YOGA FOR BEGINNERS; EASY YOGA EXERCISES FOR ALL

ZIKA IKOKU

ISBN-13: 9798335825801
ISBN-10: 1477123456

Cover design by: Art Painter
Library of Congress Control Number: 2018675309
Printed in the United States of America

TABLE OF CONTENTS

Embracing the journey and the benefits of a lifelong yoga practice

Appendix

Introduction

If you are want to start yoga but aren't sure what to do .This is a very comprehensive book of the ins and outs of Yoga, all its benefits, and various exercises to carry out for different people to improve their health. It goes in depth in explaining the different yoga exercises done for people in different walks of life. Looking to relax? Looking to get in better shape? Are you pregnant? This book will certainly improve your current living standard.

Chapter 1: Understanding Yoga

Here is your comprehensive guide to starting a life-changing yoga practice: Yoga for Beginners. . This book aims to give you an accessible and understandable introduction to yoga giving you the skills and information you need to begin and maintain a rewarding practice.

Yoga: A Brief Overview and Its Origins.

Yoga offers a comprehensive approach to wellbeing and has roots dating back over 5000 years into Indias ancient traditions. Yoga is about achieving harmony between the mind, body and spirit. The word yuj comes from the Sanskrit word yuj which means to unite. . The rich spiritual philosophical and physical traditions of Buddhism Jainism and Hinduism have all been incorporated into the practice as it has developed over time. Yoga is practiced in many different forms across the globe today and each one adds to the wide range of methods and approaches that support people in finding balance and developing personally.

The Advantages of Yoga Exercise.

 Doing yoga has a profound effect on your body and mind. Yoga promotes general health and vitality while improving physical strength flexibility and balance. Its an exercise regimen that incorporates breathing exercises relaxation methods and mindful movement that goes beyond conventional exercise. Yoga is well known for its capacity to improve focus lessen stress and foster emotional stability. Through the integration of physical and mental health yoga facilitates a more equilibrium and focused existence enabling you to handle everyday responsibilities with increased comfort and adaptability.

What this book will likely contain.

You'll take a methodical approach to learning yoga with Yoga for Beginners which will walk you through every facet of the discipline. Chapter 1 of the book Understanding Yoga provides an overview of the philosophy history and different forms of yoga in addition to outlining its core advantages. You will learn how to set up the ideal practice area recognize your bodys needs and become proficient with basic breathing techniques in Chapter 2: Setting Up for Your Yoga Practice. You will learn the fundamental standing sitting lying and balancing poses in Chapter 3: Foundational Yoga Poses. Each pose is accompanied by comprehensive instructions to ensure your safety and effectiveness. You can find instructions on designing a customized yoga routine adding new poses and monitoring your progress in Chapter 4: Building a Routine. Yoga for Different Needs Chapter 5 offers focused practices for stress relief flexibility strength and more. It also addresses particular conditions and goals. In order to improve your yoga journey overall Chapter 6: Developing a Mindful Practice delves into the integration of intention and meditation. Lastly Chapter 7: Overcoming Common Challenges offers helpful guidance on how to handle discomfort maintain motivation and get past typical roadblocks. Regardless of your yoga experience level this book provides a helpful and enlightening route to realizing the numerous advantages of yoga. Yoga for Beginners is your reliable guide on the path to a healthier more balanced life because it offers straightforward directions useful advice and a sympathetic approach.

Chapter 2: Preparing for Your Yoga Practice

ELearning poses and sequences is not the only thing that comes with starting a yoga journey. Setting up your physical space and yourself physically is crucial to getting the most out of your practice. This chapter will walk you through creating a cozy and intentional yoga space becoming aware of your body's needs and learning the basics of breathing exercises.

1. **Setting Up a Yoga Room.** Creating a Cozy and Committed Area. Organizing your home to be a yoga space can improve your practice significantly. This doesnt necessarily mean you need a big space but it should be somewhere you feel comfortable and free to move around. Here are some pointers for arranging your yoga area:. Pick a Quiet Area: Make your choice in a location that is largely free of noise and distractions. Youll be able to concentrate and unwind during your practice in a quieter setting. Make Sure You Have Enough Room: You must have enough space to comfortably extend your arms and legs. Make sure you have enough room to adjust into different poses without risk. Incorporate Personal Touches: Arrange your furnishings in a way that promotes equilibrium and serenity within you. Items such as candles plants or calming colors may fall under this category. Basic Tools. Acquiring a few essential pieces of equipment can improve your work and help you learn. These are

the necessities:. Yoga Mat: Traction and cushioning are features of a high-quality yoga mat. Select one that fits comfortably under your hands and feet and provides adequate grip. Yoga blocks: When you need additional support in a pose blocks can help with alignment and balance. They can also help make some poses easier to achieve. Yoga Strap: Using a strap will help you stretch and align yourself properly. Reaching and maintaining flexible poses is where it really shines. Blanket: A blanket can serve as a prop in restorative techniques as extra padding or as support when doing seated poses.

2. **Recognizing Your Body.** Basics of Anatomy Relevant to Yoga. Its possible to practice yoga safely and effectively if you have a basic anatomy understanding. Here are some essential ideas:. Major muscle groups including the quadriceps hamstrings and core muscles should be familiar to you. You can engage and stretch these muscles more effectively if you understand how they function. Alignment and Joints: Observe how your joints such as the hips knees and shoulders feel in different positions. For every pose to have its full benefits and to avoid strain alignment is key. Preventing injuries and Paying Attention to Your Body Are Important. Yoga emphasizes self-awareness and body awareness above all else. Heres how to guarantee a secure procedure:. Respect Your Limits: Finding balance rather than pushing yourself to the edge is the goal of yoga. Adjust as necessary and back off if a pose causes you pain or discomfort. Employ Props: To

enhance the accessibility and comfort of poses dont be afraid to use props like blocks and straps. They can assist you in preserving appropriate alignment and avoiding strain. Consult a Professional: To customize your practice to your needs if you have any pre-existing conditions or injuries you should think about speaking with a certified yoga instructor or your healthcare provider.

3. Methods of Inhalation. An overview of breath control or pranayama. A key component of yoga is breath control or pranayama which enhances focus and relaxation and complements physical postures. To get you going consider these fundamental methods:. Diaphragmatic breathing sometimes referred to as belly breathing is a breathing technique in which your abdomen contracts during exhalation and expands during inhalation. This facilitates diaphragm engagement and expands lung capacity. Box breathing involves four counts: four counts of inhalation four counts of holding the breath four counts of exhalation and four counts of holding the breath out. This method aids in enhancing focus and calming the nervous system. Nadi Shodhana or alternate nostril breathing involves closing one nostril with your thumb inhaling through the other closing it again and exhaling through the first nostril. Change your nose several times in a row. This exercise helps to improve mental clarity and energy balance in the body. Start with Easy Breathing Exercises. These breathing techniques can help you center yourself and improve your experience as a whole. Sama Vritti or equal breathing involves taking equal amounts of time to inhale and exhale. This produces a calming atmosphere and a steady rhythm. Breathe in for four counts hold it for seven counts and then release it for eight counts. This technique is known as 4-7-8. This method works particularly well for relieving tension and promoting relaxation. Setting up a space where you feel safe and at ease learning about your body and becoming proficient with basic breathing exercises are all important aspects of getting ready for a yoga practice. You can create a solid foundation for an enjoyable and long-lasting yoga practice by arranging your practice area thoughtfully paying attention to your bodys cues and using mindful breathing.

Chapter 3: Basic Yoga Poses

The foundational poses of yoga that form the basis of your practice will be covered in this chapter. These positions can be divided into four categories: standing sitting lying down and balancing. You can improve your strength flexibility and balance by learning these fundamental poses which will also help you get ready for more difficult ones.

1. Standing Poses
Standing poses are essential for building strength and stability. They engage multiple muscle groups and improve overall balance. Here are some key standing poses to incorporate into your practice. Posing in a standing position. To increase your strength and stability you must practice standing poses. They increase overall balance and work a variety of muscle groups.:

"Mountain Pose" (Tadasana)

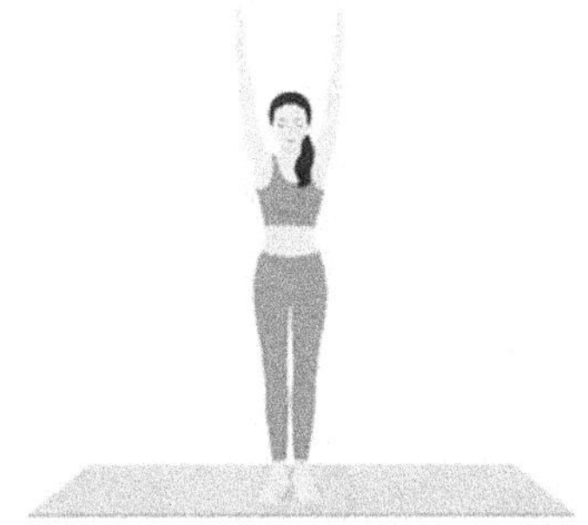

How to Do It: Stand with your feet together, or hip-width apart if more comfortable. Distribute your weight evenly across both feet. Engage your thighs, lift your chest, and lengthen your spine. Relax your shoulders away from your ears and keep your arms at your sides with palms facing forward. Gaze straight ahead.
Benefits: Improves posture, strengthens thighs and core, and enhances balance and stability.

"Downward-Facing Dog" (Adho Mukha Svanasana)

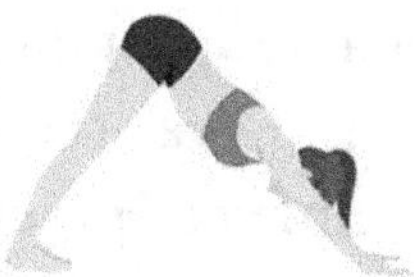

How to Do It: Start on your hands and knees. Spread your fingers wide and press firmly into the mat. Lift your hips up and back, straightening your legs as much as possible. Your body should form an inverted "V" shape. Keep your feet hip-width apart and your hands shoulder-width apart. Press your heels toward the floor.
Benefits: Stretches the hamstrings, calves, and spine, strengthens the arms and legs, and improves circulation.

"Warrior I" (Virabhadrasana I)

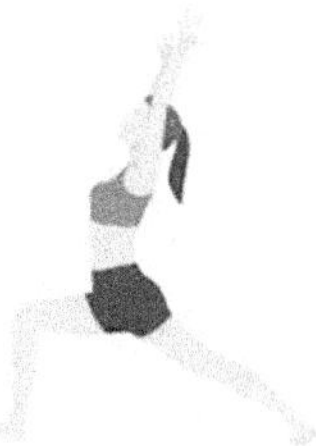

How to Do It: Step one foot back and bend the front knee, ensuring it is directly over your ankle. Keep your back leg straight and your toes pointing forward. Raise your arms overhead, palms facing each other, and lift your chest. Gaze forward.
Benefits: Strengthens the legs, opens the hips and chest, and improves focus and balance.

"Warrior II" (Virabhadrasana II)

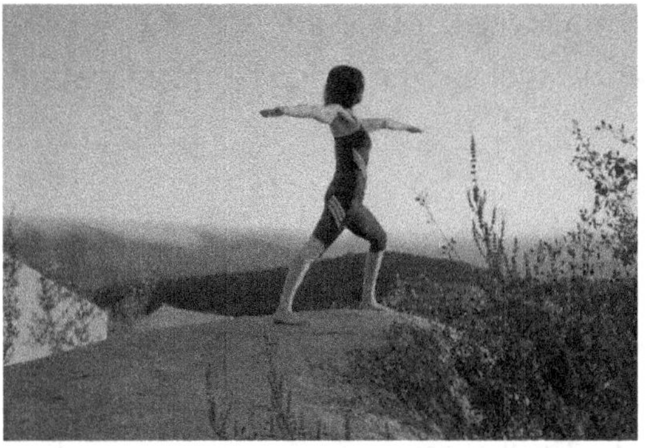

How to Do It: From Warrior I, open your hips and shoulders to face the side, extending your arms parallel to the floor, palms down. Gaze over your front hand. Keep your front knee bent and your back leg straight.
Benefits: Strengthens the legs, opens the hips and chest, and increases stamina and concentration.

"Tree Pose "(Vrksasana)

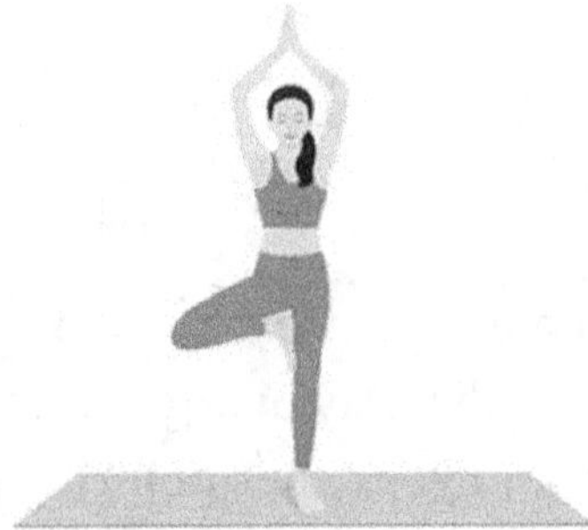

How to Do It: Stand on one leg and place the sole of your other foot against the inner thigh or calf (avoid the knee). Bring your hands together at your chest or extend them overhead. Focus on a fixed point in front of you to maintain balance.
Benefits: Improves balance and stability, strengthens the legs and core, and enhances concentration.

2. Seated Poses
Seated poses are great for stretching and relaxing. They help to improve flexibility and calm the mind. Here are some essential seated poses:

"Easy Pose" (Sukhasana)

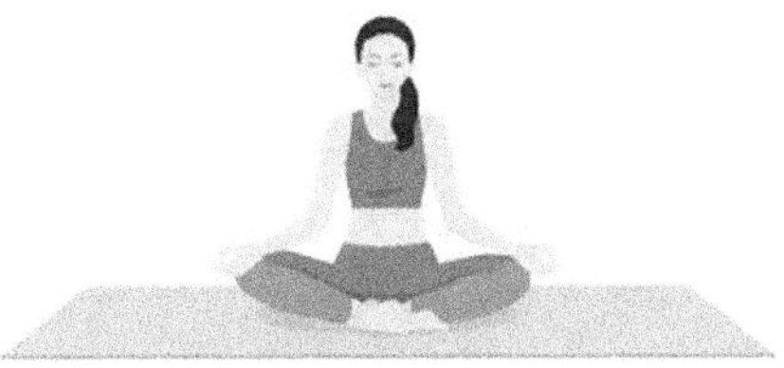

How to Do It: Sit with your legs crossed comfortably in front of you. Keep your spine straight and shoulders relaxed. Rest your hands on your knees with palms facing up or down. Close your eyes and focus on your breath.
Benefits: Calms the mind, opens the hips, and improves posture.

"Forward Fold" (Paschimottanasana)

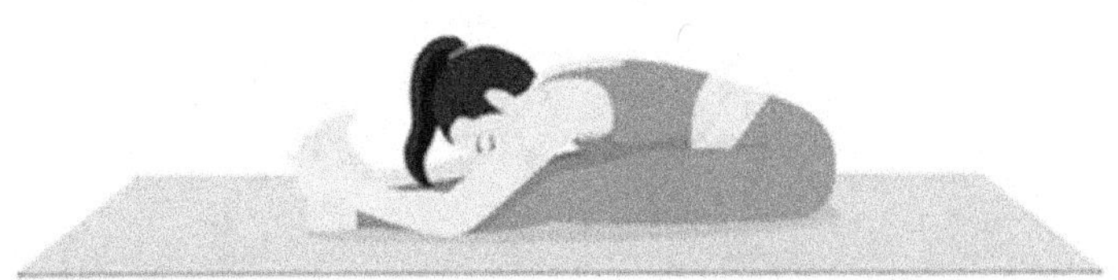

How to Do It: Sit with your legs extended straight in front of you. Inhale to lengthen your spine, and exhale as you reach forward, aiming to hold your feet or shins. Keep your back as straight as possible.
Benefits: Stretches the hamstrings, lower back, and spine, and helps to calm the nervous system.

"Seated Twist" (Ardha Matsyendrasana)

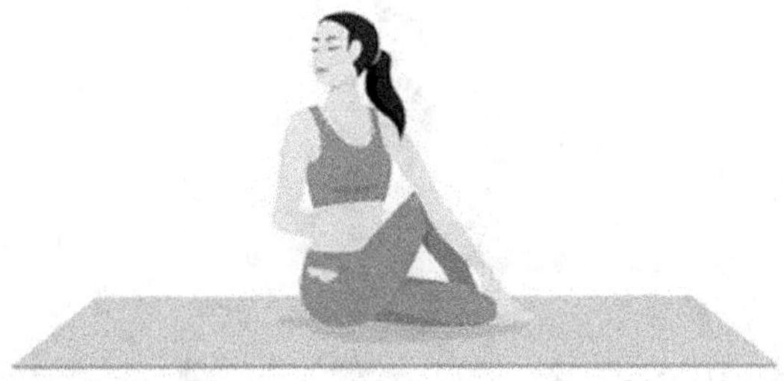

How to Do It: Sit with your legs extended. Bend one knee and place the foot on the opposite side of your thigh. Twist your torso toward the bent knee, placing your opposite elbow outside the knee. Hold the twist and then switch sides.
Benefits: Increases spinal flexibility, massages abdominal organs, and aids digestion.

3. Lying Down Poses
Lying down poses are excellent for relaxation and gentle stretching. They help in cooling down after a practice and can be very restorative:

"Corpse Pose" (Savasana)

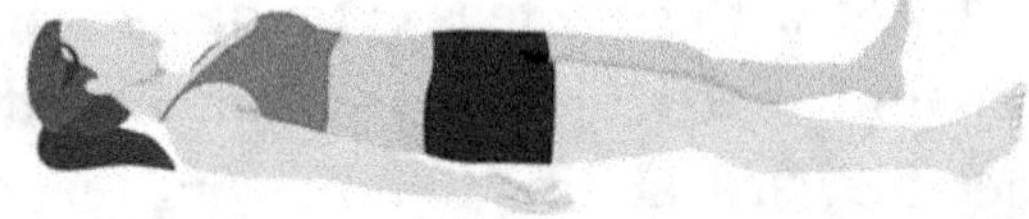

How to Do It: Lie flat on your back with your legs extended and arms relaxed at your sides, palms facing

up. Close your eyes and focus on your breath, allowing
your body to fully relax.
Benefits: Promotes relaxation and mental clarity,
reduces stress, and calms the nervous system.

"Bridge Pose" (Setu Bandhasana)

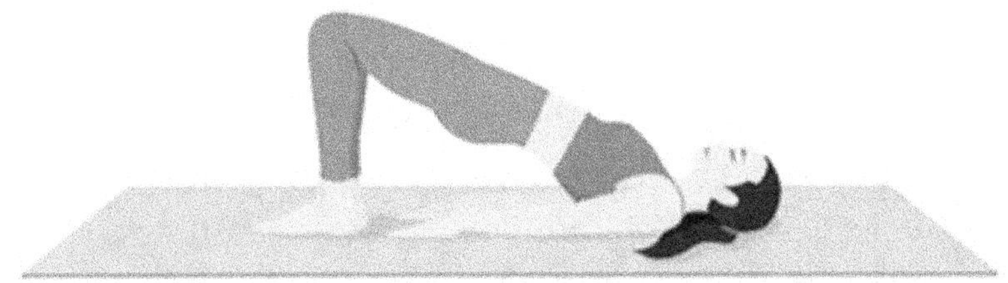

How to Do It: Lie on your back with your knees bent
and feet hip-width apart. Press your feet into the mat
and lift your hips towards the ceiling. Clasp your hands
under your back and press your arms into the floor.
Hold the pose and then lower your hips.
Benefits: Strengthens the back, glutes, and legs, opens
the chest and hips, and stimulates the abdominal
organs.

"Legs-Up-The-Wall Pose" (Viparita Karani)

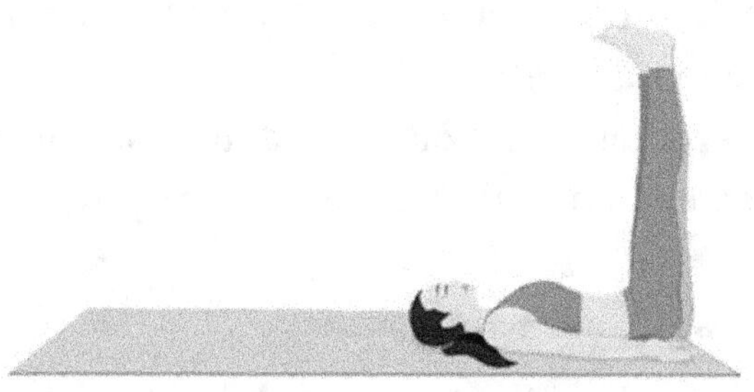

How to Do It: Sit next to a wall and lie on your back. Swing your legs up the wall while keeping your hips as close to the wall as comfortable. Rest your arms at your sides and focus on deep, even breathing. Benefits: Relieves tired legs and feet, improves circulation, and calms the mind.

4. Balancing Poses
Balancing poses challenge your stability and coordination, helping to strengthen your core and improve focus:

"Tabletop Pose" (Bharmanasana)

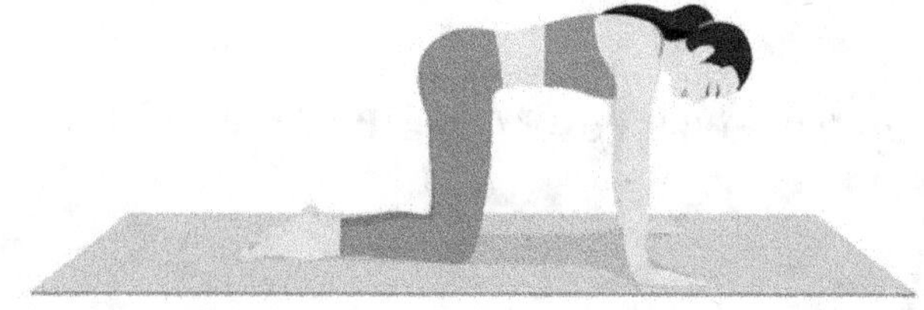

How to Do It: Start on your hands and knees, with wrists directly under shoulders and knees under hips. Engage your core and keep your back flat. This pose serves as a foundation for many other poses.

Benefits: Strengthens the core, improves spinal alignment, and prepares you for more complex poses.

"Child's Pose" (Balasana)

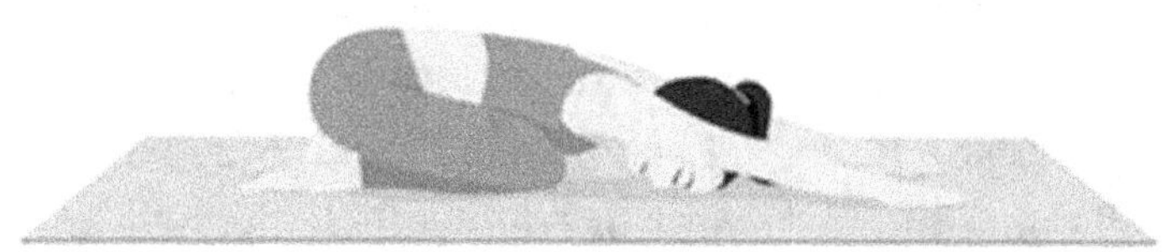

How to Do It: From a kneeling position, sit back on your heels and extend your arms forward, lowering your torso towards the floor. Rest your forehead on the mat and breathe deeply.
Benefits: Stretches the back, hips, and thighs, calms the mind, and provides a gentle rest.

"Cat-Cow Pose" (Marjaryasana-Bitilasana)

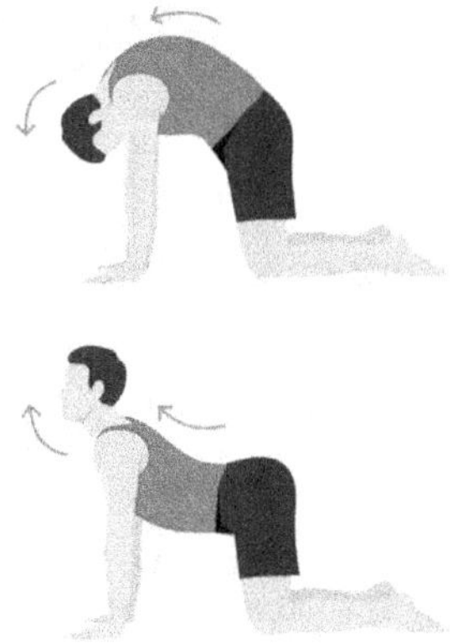

How to Do It: Start on your hands and knees. Inhale as you arch your back (Cow Pose), lifting your head and tailbone. Exhale as you round your spine (Cat Pose), tucking your chin and pelvis. Flow between these positions with your breath.

Benefits: Increases spinal flexibility, warms up the body, and relieves back tension.

By incorporating these basic poses into your practice, you will build a strong foundation for further exploration in yoga. Each pose offers unique benefits and contributes to your overall well-being, helping you develop strength, flexibility, and balance both physically and mentally.

Chapter 4: Building a Routine

CEstablishing a Schedule. To truly benefit from your yoga practice and incorporate it into your life you must establish a regular yoga routine. This chapter will cover how to create a beginners yoga routine that fits your individual objectives how to efficiently organize your practice and how to advance your practice over time.

1. Putting Together a Yoga Practice for Beginners. How to Start Your Practice. Its crucial to begin as a beginner with a routine that fits your goals and is

doable. Heres a quick guide to making your own routine:. Take It Slowly: Start with three to four sessions of fifteen to thirty minutes each. You can develop a habit like this without getting overwhelmed. Pick Your Priority: Prioritize relaxation flexibility or strength during each practice session. This aids in routine organization and goal achievement. Warm-Up and Cool-Down: Use a quick warm-up to get your body ready for exercise and afterward a cool-down to unwind and replenish. An example of a routine structure. Warm-up for five minutes. Warm up your body with some gentle stretches or breathing techniques. primary practice (15–20 minutes). Pick four to six poses that correspond with your daily focus (e. g. G. an assortment of seated standing and balance positions). Allow to cool down (5 minutes). Stretches or relaxation positions can aid in your bodys healing.

2. **Example Plans for Various Objectives.** To reduce stress:. Begin with the Childs Pose (Balasana) and move into the Cat-Cow Pose (Marjaryasana-Bitilasana). Main Practice:. Dog With His Back to the Sun (Adho Mukha Svanasana). Veteran No. 2 (Virabhadrasana II). Forward-Leaning Position (Paschimottanasana). Pose with your legs up the wall (Viparita Karani). Cool-down: Deep breathing techniques and the corpse pose or savasana. For adaptability:. Warm-up: Sun Salutations or Dynamic Stretches. Main Practice:. The Mountain Pose (Tadasana) and the Tree Pose (Vrksasana). Twist while sitting (Ardha Matsyendrasana). Folding forward

(Paschimottanasana). Pose of Bridge (Setu Bandhasana). Cool-down: Light stretches with an emphasis on the worked areas. For Power:. Warm-up: Dynamic stretching or Sun Salutations. Main Practice:. Virtuabhadrasana I or Warrior I. Adho Mukha Svanasana or the downward-facing dog. Plank Pose (Kumbhakasana): For extra strength do this optionally. Holding Bridge Pose (Setu Bandhasana). Practice deep breathing techniques and Childs Pose (Balasana) as a cool-down.

3. How Your Practice Should Be Organized. Establishing a Reliable Schedule. Frequency: Aim for regular sessions ideally 3-4 times a week to establish a habit and see progress. Duration: Start with manageable durations (15-30 minutes) and gradually increase as you build endurance and confidence. Variety: Mix different types of poses and routines to keep your practice engaging and address different aspects of fitness. Creating a Balanced Practice. Include Different Pose Types: Incorporate standing seated lying down and balancing poses to ensure a well-rounded practice. Focus on Breath: Integrate breathing techniques throughout your routine to enhance relaxation and effectiveness. Listen to Your Body: Adjust the intensity and duration of your practice based on how your body feels.

4. How to Progress. Introducing New Poses and Variations. Start with Basics: Once you're comfortable with basic poses start exploring variations and more advanced poses gradually. Incorporate New

Techniques: Add new breathing techniques or sequences to challenge yourself and keep your practice dynamic. Seek Guidance: Consider taking classes or following online tutorials to learn proper techniques and new poses. Setting Realistic Goals and Tracking Progress. Set Specific Goals: Define clear achievable goals such as improving flexibility mastering a new pose or increasing practice frequency. Track Your Progress: Keep a journal or use an app to record your practice sessions note improvements and reflect on how you feel. Celebrate Achievements: Recognize and celebrate milestones no matter how small. This will help keep you motivated and positive. Adapting Your Routine. Modify as Needed: Be flexible with your routine based on your progress and any changes in your physical or mental state. Reassess Goals: Periodically reassess your goals and adjust your practice to ensure it remains aligned with your evolving needs and interests. Building a yoga routine involves thoughtful planning and consistency. By setting up a structured approach incorporating a variety of poses and regularly reassessing your goals you can create a fulfilling and effective practice that supports your growth and well-being. Embrace the journey and remember that progress in yoga is a personal and ongoing process.

Chapter 5: Yoga for Different Needs

Yoga is a versatile practice that can be tailored to meet various needs and goals. In this chapter we will explore how to adapt yoga practices for stress relief flexibility strength and specific conditions. By understanding how to focus your practice on these different aspects you can effectively address your individual needs and enhance your overall well-being.

1. Yoga for Stress Relief. Poses and Practices for Relaxation. For stress relief and relaxation yoga has been shown to be an effective tool. You can help relax the body and mind by incorporating particular poses and techniques into your practice. Balasana also known as Childs Pose is a mild resting pose that eases nervous system tension and releases hip and back tension. The forward fold also known as paschimottanasana eases lower back and hamstring strains while fostering calmness. Legs Up the Wall Pose (Viparita Karani): This balancing pose promotes better circulation and lowers stress levels. Corpse Pose (Savasana): Unwind thoroughly and incorporate the advantages of your practice with this profoundly calming pose. Including meditation and mindfulness. Include mindfulness and meditation in your daily routine to improve stress relief even more:. Breathing with awareness: To relax the body and mind concentrate on taking slow deep breaths. Particularly useful breathing techniques include box breathing and diaphragmatic breathing. Meditation with a guide: To help you relax and concentrate try guided meditations. A variety of stress-reduction-focused meditation techniques are available through apps and internet resources. Body Scan Meditation: This technique helps you relax and relieve stress by focusing your attention on various body parts.

2. **Yoga**: The Art of Flexibility. Increase Your Flexibility with These Stretches and Poses. Your range of motion will be improved and your risk of injury will be decreased with increased flexibility. Stretches and poses like these can help you become more flexible. Adho Mukha Svanasana (Downward-Facing Dog): Increases overall flexibility by stretching the calves hamstrings and spine. Seated Forward Fold (Paschimottanasana): Targets the hamstrings and lower back deepening the stretch over time. Butterfly Pose (Baddha Konasana): Opens the hips and groin promoting flexibility in the lower body. Cobra Pose (Bhujangasana): Stretches the chest and spine enhancing flexibility in the back. Tips for Safe and Effective Stretching. Warm-Up First: Always warm up your muscles with gentle movement before stretching to prevent injury. Avoid Overstretching: Stretch to the point of mild discomfort not pain. Overstretching can lead to injuries. Use Props: Utilize yoga blocks straps and blankets to assist in reaching and maintaining poses. Breathe Deeply: Maintain a steady breath

throughout your stretches to deepen the pose and relax the muscles.

3. **Yoga for Strength.** Poses That Build Muscle and Endurance. Building strength through yoga enhances overall fitness and supports other physical activities. Focus on poses that engage and challenge your muscles:. Plank Pose (Kumbhakasana): Strengthens the core arms and shoulders and builds endurance. Warrior III (Virabhadrasana III): Improves balance and strengthens the legs core and back. Strengthens the legs glutes and core with Chair Pose (Utkatasana). The Boat Pose (Navasana) strengthens the core and works the abdominal muscles. Blending Yoga with Other Exercise Methods. Consider combining yoga with other exercises to enhance strength and endurance:. Cardiovascular Exercise: Activities like running cycling or swimming complement yoga by improving cardiovascular health and endurance. Strength Training: Incorporate weightlifting or resistance exercises to build muscle and support your yoga practice. Cross-Training: Engaging in various forms of exercise helps prevent overuse injuries and keeps your routine balanced.

4. **Yoga for Specific Conditions.** Adapting Poses for Common Issues. Yoga can be adapted to address specific conditions and physical issues. Here's how to modify poses to accommodate common concerns:. For back pain try poses like Childs Pose (Balasana) and Cat-Cow Pose (Marjaryasana-Bitilasana) to gently

stretch and strengthen the back. Stay away from high-impact positions and deep backbends. Tight Hips: To increase flexibility and release tension in the hip flexors try incorporating poses like Pigeon Pose (Eka Pada Rajakapotasana) and Butterfly Pose (Baddha Konasana). Knee Pain: To prevent making your knee pain worse choose poses that have a milder impact such as seated stretches and encouraged warrior poses. Making Adjustments and Using Props for Various Needs. Yoga is beneficial and accessible for a range of needs thanks to props and modifications. Yoga blocks: Support and aid in alignment when performing standing poses. They can also be used to adjust poses to make them more comfortable. Yoga Straps: Assist in reaching and holding poses especially useful for stretches and maintaining proper alignment. Bolsters and Blankets: Offer support in restorative poses and provide cushioning for added comfort. You can improve your well-being and accomplish your objectives by customizing your yoga practice to meet particular needs such as stress relief flexibility strength or managing particular conditions. Modifications and pose adaptations guarantee that yoga is a safe and beneficial practice for all.

Chapter 6: Developing a Mindful Practice

As you continue your journey into yoga youll find that the practice is about much more than just physical postures. Yoga is a holistic practice that encompasses the mind body and spirit. One of the most powerful tools you can incorporate into your yoga routine is mindfulness especially through meditation. In this chapter well explore how to develop a mindful practice by incorporating meditation understanding its basics and setting intentions that can enhance your overall yoga experience.

1. Incorporating Meditation. Meditation is a natural extension of yoga and plays a crucial role in deepening your practice. While yoga helps to align the body and breath meditation focuses on calming the mind and cultivating inner peace. By integrating meditation into your yoga routine you can enhance your mental clarity reduce stress and develop a greater sense of self-awareness. Incorporating meditation doesnt have to be complicated. You can start with just a few minutes of focused breathing at the beginning or end of your yoga session. Over time as you become more comfortable you can extend the duration and explore different meditation techniques that resonate with you.

2. **Basics of Meditation and Mindfulness.** Mindfulness is the practice of being fully present in the moment aware of your thoughts feelings and surroundings without judgment. Meditation is a key practice that helps cultivate mindfulness. By regularly practicing meditation you can train your mind to stay focused calm and centered. At its core meditation involves sitting quietly and focusing your attention on a single point of reference such as your breath a mantra or even a specific part of your body. The goal is not to empty your mind of all thoughts but rather to observe them without attachment and gently bring your focus back to your point of reference whenever your mind wanders.

3. **Simple Meditation Techniques to Complement Your Yoga Practice.** There are many meditation techniques that you can easily incorporate into your yoga practice. Here are a few simple methods to get you started:. Focused Breathing: Sit in a comfortable position and close your eyes. Take slow deep breaths focusing all your attention on the sensation of the breath entering and leaving your body. If your mind starts to wander gently bring your focus back to your breath. Body Scan Meditation: Lie down in Savasana (Corpse Pose) at the end of your yoga practice. Starting from the top of your head slowly scan down through your body bringing awareness to each part. Notice any areas of tension and consciously relax them. Mantra Meditation: Choose a word or phrase (mantra) that resonates with you such as peace or I am calm. Repeat

this mantra silently to yourself during meditation allowing it to anchor your thoughts and bring you into a state of tranquility. Loving-Kindness Meditation: Begin by focusing on your breath. Then gradually bring to mind someone you care about and silently wish them happiness health and peace. Expand these wishes to others in your life including yourself. This meditation fosters compassion and positive emotions.

4. The Role of Intention. In yoga intention or Sankalpa is a powerful tool that can guide your practice and your life. Creating an intention is similar to sowing a seed in your mind that develops and affects your perception behavior and experiences as a whole. Intentions are more about the present and how you want to approach your practice or life in general than goals which are frequently specific and focused on the future. For instance you may want to practice self-acceptance kindness or patience during a yoga session. By establishing an intention you establish a mental framework that directs your work and keeps you concentrated on your priorities. 5. Organizing Your Practice with Intentions. Spend a few minutes at the start of your yoga practice thinking about what you want to bring into your practice to set an intention. Take a few deep breaths close your eyes and ask yourself What do I need today? or What quality do I want to cultivate? You could even make it as simple as I will practice gratitude or I will listen to my body. . . As you move through your yoga poses keep your intention in mind. If your mind starts to wander or if you encounter a challenging pose gently remind yourself of your intention. This can help you stay present and connected to your practice. 6. How Intention Enhances Your Overall Yoga Experience. When you practice yoga with intention you bring a deeper level of awareness and meaning to your practice. Intentions help you stay focused centered and aligned with your inner values. They can also provide a sense of purpose and motivation especially on days when you might feel less inspired to practice. By regularly setting and reflecting on your intentions youll find that your yoga practice becomes more than just a physical exercise it becomes a powerful tool for personal growth and transformation. Over time youll notice that the intentions you set on your mat start to influence your life off the mat helping you live with more mindfulness compassion and clarity. Incorporating meditation and setting intentions are essential aspects of developing a mindful yoga practice. As you continue on your yoga journey remember that the true essence of yoga lies not just in the physical poses but in the mindfulness intention and inner awareness that you cultivate along the way.

Chapter 7: Overcoming Common Challenges

As you continue your journey into yoga youll find that the practice is about much more than just physical postures. Yoga is a holistic practice that encompasses the mind body and spirit. One of the most powerful tools you can incorporate into your yoga routine is mindfulness especially through meditation. In this chapter well explore how to develop a mindful practice by incorporating meditation understanding its basics and setting intentions that can enhance your overall yoga experience.

1. Incorporating Meditation. Meditation is a natural extension of yoga and plays a crucial role in deepening your practice. While yoga helps to align the body and breath meditation focuses on calming the mind and cultivating inner peace. By integrating meditation into your yoga routine you can enhance your mental clarity reduce stress and develop a greater sense of self-awareness. Incorporating meditation doesnt have to be complicated. You can start with just a few minutes of focused breathing at the beginning or end of your yoga session. Over time as you become more comfortable you can extend the duration and explore different meditation techniques that resonate with you.

2. **Basics of Meditation and Mindfulness.** Mindfulness is the practice of being fully present in the moment aware of your thoughts feelings and surroundings without judgment. Meditation is a key practice that helps cultivate mindfulness. By regularly practicing meditation you can train your mind to stay focused calm and centered. At its core meditation involves sitting quietly and focusing your attention on a single point of reference such as your breath a mantra or even a specific part of your body. The goal is not to empty your mind of all thoughts but rather to observe them without attachment and gently bring your focus back to your point of reference whenever your mind wanders.

3. **Simple Meditation Techniques to Complement Your Yoga Practice.** There are many meditation techniques that you can easily incorporate into your yoga practice. Here are a few simple methods to get you started:. Focused Breathing: Sit in a comfortable position and close your eyes. Take slow deep breaths focusing all your attention on the sensation of the breath entering and leaving your body. If your mind starts to wander gently bring your focus back to your breath. Body Scan Meditation: Lie down in Savasana (Corpse Pose) at the end of your yoga practice. Starting from the top of your head slowly scan down through your body bringing awareness to each part. Notice any areas of tension and consciously relax them. Mantra Meditation: Choose a word or phrase (mantra) that resonates with you such as peace or I am calm. Repeat

this mantra silently to yourself during meditation allowing it to anchor your thoughts and bring you into a state of tranquility. Loving-Kindness Meditation: Begin by focusing on your breath. Then gradually bring to mind someone you care about and silently wish them happiness health and peace. Expand these wishes to others in your life including yourself. This meditation fosters compassion and positive emotions.

4. The Role of Intention. In yoga intention or Sankalpa is a powerful tool that can guide your practice and your life. Creating an intention is similar to sowing a seed in your mind that develops and affects your perception behavior and experiences as a whole. Intentions are more about the present and how you want to approach your practice or life in general than goals which are frequently specific and focused on the future. For instance you may want to practice self-acceptance kindness or patience during a yoga session. By establishing an intention you establish a mental framework that directs your work and keeps you concentrated on your priorities.

5. Organizing Your Practice with Intentions. Spend a few minutes at the start of your yoga practice thinking about what you want to bring into your practice to set an intention. Take a few deep breaths close your eyes and ask yourself What do I need today? or What quality do I want to cultivate? You could even make it as simple as I will practice gratitude or I will listen to my body. . . As you move through your yoga poses keep your intention in mind. If your mind starts to wander

or if you encounter a challenging pose gently remind yourself of your intention. This can help you stay present and connected to your practice.

6. How Intention Enhances Your Overall Yoga Experience. When you practice yoga with intention you bring a deeper level of awareness and meaning to your practice. Intentions help you stay focused centered and aligned with your inner values. They can also provide a sense of purpose and motivation especially on days when you might feel less inspired to practice. By regularly setting and reflecting on your intentions youll find that your yoga practice becomes more than just a physical exercise it becomes a powerful tool for personal growth and transformation. Over time youll notice that the intentions you set on your mat start to influence your life off the mat helping you live with more mindfulness compassion and clarity. Incorporating meditation and setting intentions are essential aspects of developing a mindful yoga practice. As you continue on your yoga journey remember that the true essence of yoga lies not just in the physical poses but in the mindfulness intention and inner awareness that you cultivate along the way.

Conclusion: Your Yoga Journey Ahead

Yoga is more than just a physical practice it's a lifelong journey of self-discovery growth and transformation. As you continue on this path you'll find that yoga has the potential to touch every aspect of your life—body mind and spirit. The journey ahead is filled with opportunities to deepen your practice explore new styles and integrate the principles of yoga into your daily life. Stay Open to Learning: As you progress remain open to learning and trying new things. Explore different styles of yoga attend workshops or delve into yoga philosophy. Each new experience will add richness to your practice. Honor Your Progress: Take time to reflect on how far you've come. Enjoy your accomplishments and use them as inspiration to keep moving forward whether they are improved flexibility a stronger bond with your breath or an increased sense of calm. As your practice develops think about establishing new goals for yourself on the journey. These could be practicing more advanced poses going deeper into meditation or incorporating yoga into your everyday routine.

2. Promotion of Ongoing Practice and Research. A fruitful yoga practice requires consistency. Even though the road may not always be smooth sailing the rewards of consistent practice make the effort

worthwhile. Keep Showing Up: The most important thing you can do for your practice is to keep showing up on your mat. Even on days when you don't feel like practicing remember that yoga is there to support you in every stage of life. Explore Beyond the Mat: Yoga doesn't end when you roll up your mat. Explore how the principles of yoga such as mindfulness compassion and non-attachment can be applied in your daily life. The more you integrate yoga into your life the more you'll experience its transformative power. Discover Joy in the Journey: The goal of yoga is to discover joy in the process rather than to attain perfection. Savor every second of your practice whether its a difficult pose or a quiet period.

3. Resources for Additional Education. You might want to look into other resources as you proceed with your yoga journey in order to improve your knowledge and technique. These suggestions are as follows:. Books:. The Heart of Yoga by T. K. V. Desikachar: A comprehensive guide to the philosophy and practice of yoga offering insights into the traditional teachings of yoga. Light on Yoga by B. K. S. Iyengar: A well-known manual that offers thorough directions and pictures for hundreds of yoga positions. A key text for comprehending the philosophical underpinnings of yoga is Sri Swami Satchidanandas Patanjali Yoga Sutras. Online Courses:. Yoga with Adriene: A well-known YouTube channel that specializes in mindfulness and self-care and offers free yoga classes for practitioners of all skill levels. Glo: An online resource offering meditation Pilates and a variety of yoga classes ranging from beginner to advanced. In addition to strength training and mindfulness exercises Alo Moves provides a range of yoga classes such as Hatha Vinyasa and restorative yoga. Neighborhood Studios:. Find a Local Studio: In-person yoga classes at a nearby studio can offer individualized instruction and a sense of community. Seek out studios that provide workshops or classes for beginners. Workshops and Retreats: A lot of yoga studios provide workshops and retreats that concentrate on particular facets of yoga like alignment meditation or philosophy. These can be a great way to deepen your practice and connect with others.

4. Finally some wise words. Here are some parting words of wisdom to keep in mind as you continue your yoga journey:. Be Patient and Kind to Yourself: Yoga is a journey not a destination. Progress may be slow at times but every step forward is valuable. Practice self-compassion and be gentle with yourself as you grow. Trust the Process: Trust that your practice is unfolding exactly as it should. Whether you're facing challenges or enjoying a period of growth each experience is part of your unique journey. Stay Curious: Yoga is a vast and ever-evolving practice. Stay curious and open to new experiences whether it's exploring different styles trying new poses or delving into the philosophical teachings of yoga. 5. Embracing the Journey and the Benefits of a Lifelong Yoga Practice. The true beauty of yoga lies in its ability to evolve with you throughout

your life. As you embrace the journey you'll discover that yoga offers far more than physical benefits. It has the power to bring peace to your mind balance to your emotions and a deeper connection to your true self. A Lifelong Practice: From your youth to your golden years yoga is a practice that can help you at every stage of life. It adapts to your needs and grows with you providing a constant source of strength flexibility and inner peace. The Benefits Beyond the Mat: As you continue to practice you'll find that the benefits of yoga extend far beyond the mat. Whether it's greater resilience in the face of challenges a calmer mind or a deeper sense of purpose the gifts of yoga are endless. Embrace the Journey: Ultimately yoga is about embracing the journey. There will be moments of joy and moments of struggle but each step is an opportunity to learn grow and connect more deeply with yourself and the world around you. As you close this book and step forward on your yoga journey remember that you are not alone. The practice of yoga has been shared and celebrated for thousands of years and you are now part of that rich tradition. May your journey be filled with growth discovery and endless possibilities. Namaste.

Appendix:
Tips and Tricks for a
Successful Yoga Journey

As you continue your yoga journey you might find yourself seeking additional advice tips and tricks to enhance your practice. This appendix offers a collection of insights including key takeaways from the book and some new suggestions to help you get the most out of your yoga experience.

1. **Start Where You Are:** One of the most important things to remember as a beginner is to start where you are not where you think you should be. Yoga is a personal practice and everyone's journey is unique. Here are a few tips to help you embrace this mindset:. Listen to Your Body: Pay close attention to how your body feels during each pose. It's okay to modify poses or take breaks as needed. The goal is to practice safely and sustainably. Avoid Comparisons: It's easy to compare yourself to others especially in a class setting or when following online videos. Remember yoga is about your personal growth not competing with others. Be Patient: Flexibility strength and mindfulness develop over time. Celebrate small victories and be patient with your progress.

2. **Create a Dedicated Practice Space:** Having a dedicated space for your yoga practice can make it

easier to stay consistent. It doesn't have to be large or elaborate even a small corner in your home can become your yoga sanctuary. Keep It Simple: A quiet uncluttered space with enough room to stretch out on your mat is all you need. Add some calming elements like candles plants or a small altar to create a peaceful atmosphere. Eliminate Distractions: Choose a spot where you're less likely to be interrupted. Silence your phone and set aside any distractions before starting your practice. Personalize Your Space: Decorate your space with items that inspire you such as meaningful artwork crystals or a favorite piece of music. This can make your practice feel more personal and sacred.

3. Consistency Over Perfection: Consistency is key in yoga and its better to practice a little every day than to push yourself too hard in infrequent longer sessions. Short Practices Are Effective: Even a 10-minute daily practice can make a significant difference over time. Don't feel pressured to commit to an hour-long session every day. Routine Helps: Try to practice at the same time each day to build a routine. Morning practices can energize your day while evening sessions can help you unwind. Be Flexible with Your Routine: Life happens and it's okay to adjust your practice to fit your day. The important thing is to keep coming back to your mat.

4. Embrace Props and Modifications: Props and modifications are your friends in yoga. They help you find comfort in poses deepen your stretches and ensure proper alignment. Use Blocks for Support: Yoga blocks can bring the floor closer to you in poses like

Triangle (Trikonasana) or Half Moon (Ardha Chandrasana). They're also great for seated poses where you need extra support. Straps for Flexibility: If you can't reach your feet in poses like Seated Forward Fold (Paschimottanasana) use a yoga strap to bridge the gap. It allows you to maintain proper alignment while gradually increasing flexibility. Blankets for Comfort: A folded blanket can provide cushioning for your knees in poses like Low Lunge (Anjaneyasana) or support your hips in seated poses.

5. Stay Hydrated and Nourished. Yoga is a physical activity and it's important to stay hydrated and nourished to support your practice. Drink Water Before and After: Hydrate before your practice to prevent dehydration especially if you're doing a vigorous style of yoga. Drink water after your session to replenish lost fluids. Eat Light Before Practice: If you need to eat before your practice choose something light and easy to digest such as a piece of fruit or a small smoothie. Practicing on a full stomach can be uncomfortable. Post-Practice Nutrition: After your practice nourish your body with a balanced meal that includes protein healthy fats and complex carbohydrates to support recovery and energy levels.

6. Link Your Breath to Your Movement. The idea of the relationship between breath and movement is one of the core concepts of yoga. This technique also known as Vinyasa assists you in maintaining your attention and awareness. Breathe in to expand release out: Generally speaking breathe in when you are doing an expansion-focused movement such as reaching up into

Mountain Pose (Tadasana). When performing contractions or folding motions with your body such as Forward Folds release your breath. Set the Pace with Your Breath: During your practice let your breath dictate the speed. You should slow down or take a break if your breathing starts to become labored or shallow. Breath Awareness: Refocus your attention on your breathing if you notice that it has wandered. You can improve your practices mindfulness and sense of grounding by doing this small action.

7. **Blend mindfulness and meditation**: You can enhance your yoga practice by including meditation and mindfulness as we covered in Chapter 6. Start with a Few Minutes: Begin or end your practice with a few minutes of meditation. Sit in stillness concentrate on your breathing or use a mantra. Practice Mindful Movement: During your yoga session move with intention and awareness. Take note of your bodys sensation in each pose and the way your breath flows. Carry Mindfulness Off the Mat: Take the mindfulness you cultivate on the mat into your daily life. Practice being completely present whether its when youre talking eating or strolling. 8. Take Part in a Community. Finding a yoga community can provide support motivation and connection. Whether in person or online being part of a group can enrich your practice. Attend Workshops and Classes: Participating in workshops or classes either locally or online can introduce you to new practices teachers and fellow yogis. Join Online Groups: Many social media platforms have yoga groups where members share tips

challenges and experiences. Engaging with these communities can provide inspiration and encouragement. Yoga Retreats: If you're looking for a deeper experience consider attending a yoga retreat. These immersive experiences can deepen your practice and connect you with like-minded individuals. 9. Embrace the Journey. Finally remember that yoga is a lifelong journey. There's no rush to achieve a specific pose or level of flexibility. The true essence of yoga lies in the journey itself—learning growing and discovering more about yourself along the way. Be Kind to Yourself: Self-compassion is key in yoga. If you miss a practice or struggle with a pose be kind to yourself and remember that it's all part of the process. Celebrate Your Progress: Take time to acknowledge and celebrate your progress no matter how small. Each step forward is a victory on your yoga journey. Stay Curious: Keep exploring different styles poses and techniques. Yoga is a vast and rich tradition with something to offer everyone no matter where you are in your practice. These tips and tricks are here to support you as you continue your yoga journey. Whether you're a complete beginner or have been practicing for some time these insights can help you deepen your practice overcome challenges and enjoy all the benefits that yoga has to offer. Remember yoga is a personal journey and the most important thing is to enjoy the process and stay connected to your inner self.

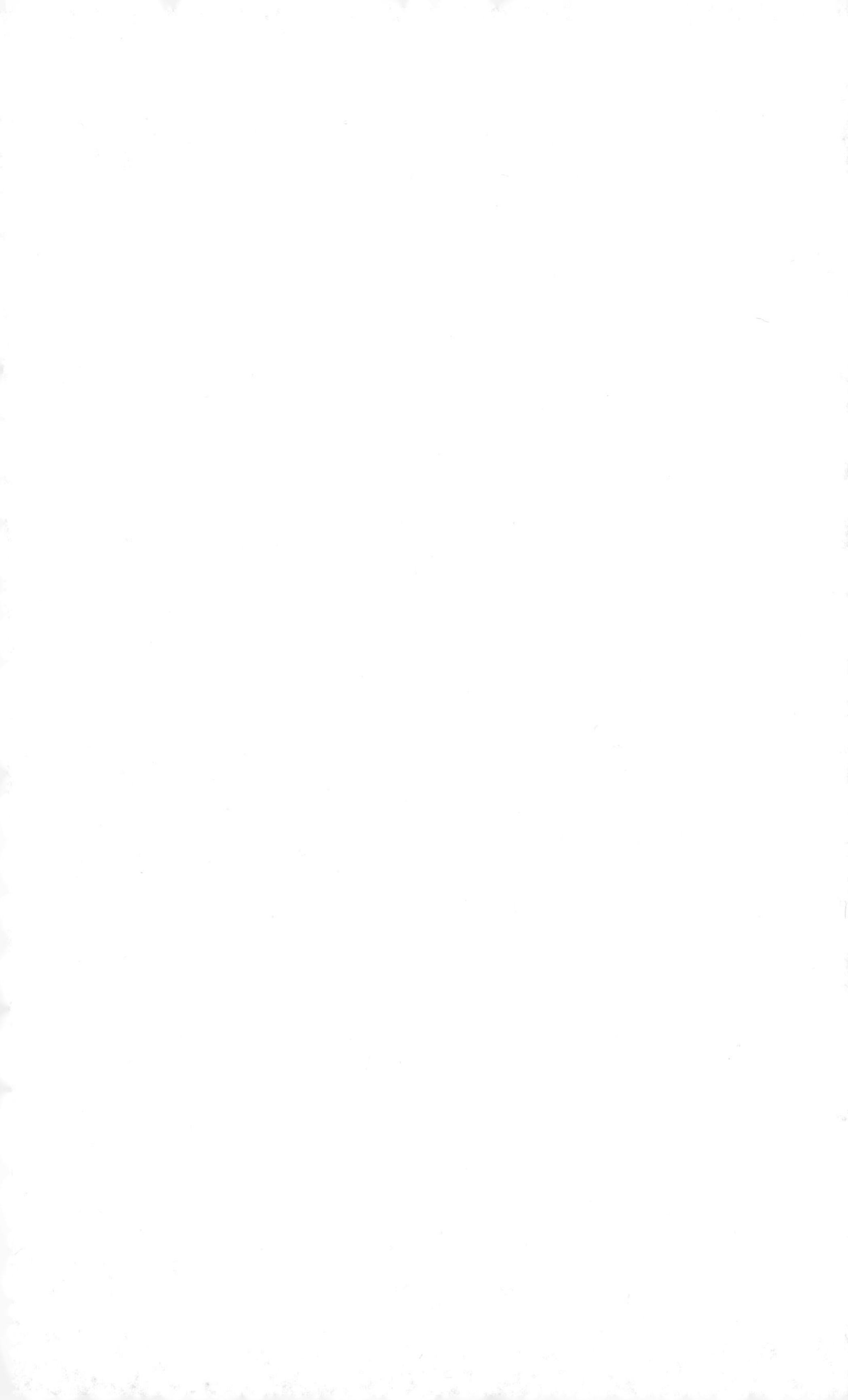

www.ingramcontent.com/pod-product-compliance
Lightning Source LLC
Chambersburg PA
CBHW051713250726